Healing Herbs
Top Must-Have Herbs With Uses and
Benifits

Table of content

Introduction...3

Chapter 1 – 5 Healing Herbs You Must Know About!.............................5

Chapter 2 – Learn About Herbs Benefits and Start Healing Yourself Naturally Today..7

Chapter 3 – Top 7 Tips To Choose Healing Herbs For Your Conditions.............11

Chapter 5 – The Power of Healing Herbs and Benefits.......................16

Conclusion 23

Introduction

Herbs have usually been used as remedies for thousands of years. Modern medicine is descended variety of previous world herbal healing techniques which have been fine-tuned and brought to research. Many of the treatments today we still use are produced directly from flowers, but their active ingredients are pure, and their therapeutic effects increased.

Though many typical healing herbs have already been overlooked for their medical benefit due to an increase of modern medicine, a lot of people are becoming aware of the hazards and side effects of some strong non-prescription medicines and are looking for a healthy alternative.

Sage is another of the healing herbs. It is a vital herb in alternative medicine due to the wide selection of diseases it has been used to treat. Sage used and may be burned in aromatherapy to help with breathing. Additionally, it may be used in tea form to reduce inflammation in the gastrointestinal tract i.e. Redness or swelling in us, as well the gums or neck upset stomach and diarrhea.

Garlic is a popular plant that's used to enable illnesses of the heart. It will also help to lower high blood pressure, reduce blood cholesterol, and reduce blood clotting. It also has antioxidant properties which operate against free radicals to decrease the chance of cancer. It has already been used to treat the virus, colds, and lung infection.

Parsley is a different one of the healing herbs. It's known to help with the prevention of kidney infections and other intestinal tract problems, including nausea and gas. You can also apply it to bug bites, reductions, and dry skin to prevent disease.

Lavender can be a healing plant that provides a gentle calming effect. It is a common tea chemical for peace, but it is also considered to aid digestion.

Strawberry leaves are another of the healing herbs usually found in teas. Like chamomile, it offers help with digestion and pleasure. It has also been applied to treat mouth, attention and neck inflammation or inflammation and it is also considered to help prevent miscarriage.

It is a number of only some of the most common healing herbs. Various tried and true herbal remedies originate from all over the world. Discovering useful herbal remedies and how to rely on them properly and properly can be very useful to your long term health. Though significant circumstances should be brought to a health care provider, many diseases could be treated with simple home remedies quickly and quickly.

Chapter 1 – 5 Healing Herbs You Must Know About!

There can be practically nothing much better than a herb to heal different problems in your body. From minor rashes around the skin to serious stomach ache, there's practically nothing that herbs cannot treat. All you need is the knowledge of various herbs and the reason of their existence. In the end, Mother Earth will not increase all those lovely things just for the cause of it; Ayurvedic doctors use diverse natural herbal products to be made by most of the herbs in the forests.

If you're preparing to buy some natural herbal products, it is important for you to know about some herbs available on our planet. Following is the number of five mostly used healing herbs that every individual should know about:

Turmeric - If you've arthritis, turmeric could be the magical solution for you. Many of the natural herbal products which are created for bone and skin -related issues include turmeric. The glowing particles of this beautiful plant become life-savers for those who proceed through the skin and mutual -related issues. It also helps in preventing Alzheimer's disease, if eaten in the proper ratio.

Cinnamon - Common in the Asian nations, a pinch of cinnamon in milk can help you save a whole lot of money. Your immune system increases and keeps you away from diverse allopathic medications, which you normally have to eat due to a cough, cool and fever. You will never have problems like diabetes and obesity if your natural products have cinnamon in them.

Ginger - Another excellent plant that grows extensively in different countries, cinnamon has a unique benefit. Add some cubes or even a portion of grated ginger in your tea and spot the decline in your stress levels. The second you take the initial glass of cinnamon tea, half of your tension vanishes in almost no time in any way! Additionally, it beats sickness.

Holy basil - Drink tea that's been created with holy basil and watch the way the tumors in your breasts, reduce in several days. Many kinds of cancers can be handled with the aid of holy basil.

Garlic - want it or not, garlic is the fact that something which will help you struggle with a whole lot of diseases. From your immune system to the constipation issue that you proceed through, there is practically nothing that garlic doesn't help you with. If you have specific minor problems, you can usually treat them every morning by eating 1 or 2 cloves of garlic. Just gulp the cloves down with water. It also helps in maintaining weight.

Chapter 2 – Learn About Herbs Benefits and Start Healing Yourself Naturally Today

Herbs benefits are something that all of us ought to be using today. Within this time of higher rates, it is comforting to know that herbs can be utilized to produce better health. Matter of fact supplement benefits is indeed good that individuals can use almost all of medical issues to heal. It does not matter if the ailment is significant or little, with a little bit of understanding you can start to rely on them today to heal your illnesses. OH, I didn't mention this yet. Nevertheless, the largest gain in using herbs is that they charge significantly less than any synthetic medicine. At the top of which they have no side effects, unlike manufactured medicines, that are impossible for the Liver to process.

Let us start our conversation about herbs gains with one of the most popular herbs, Echinacea. For a time now Echinacea has been considered a mainstream plant. Most of us know it is applied to enhance our immune system. One myth about Echinacea's immune system enhancing qualities is the fact that it just operates in the onset of a chilly. That is to date in the truth. Why would you stop taking Echinacea when your body is right at the center of fighting with an infection? Your immune system is what fights off infections, so it only produces since to reinforce your immune system the whole time it's fighting. You avoid the advancement of the infection by using Echinacea on top of a cold. Echinacea can also be used externally to help wounds or heal cuts, especially where infection occurs.

So immediately we observe that herbs benefit our excellent for our body's immune system. But there are numerous more benefits of herbs. Let us now consider the advantages to our Digestive system.

The digestive system is just one long pipe that operates from the end of our body to another. With spaces on both ends, stuff happens the other and goes in one end. It's vitally important that we keep the digestive system's areas healthy. They are open to the great and poor things we put in our body. They work in close connection to the other systems in our body, just like an immune system, the nervous system, and cardiovascular system. This means when our digestive system is doing badly it'll bring down the event of other systems. This can lead to major health problems. Here are just a couple conditions of the digestive system: Heartburn, Contamination, Ulcers, Gallstones, and Diabetes Mellitus.

Feed the areas of the digestive system so they can perform at their best constantly, and the objective of using herbs advantages is to ease, stimulate, condition. More herbs help increase the digestive system than every other system in our body.

The other supplement benefits for the digestive system are utilized for the areas of the digestive system and specific results on digestion. Like taking the plant Milk Thistle is fantastic for treating gallstones, liver problems, gallbladder, spleen, being a therapy for jaundice, varicose veins, etc. The number might continue, but I would like to speak quickly about why Milk Thistle seed extract is indeed good for the liver.

Milk Thistle extract also interferes with enterohepatic circulation. You may be asking, what does that mean? Well, toxins are constantly being moved back in forth between the liver and your intestinal tract, which means that your liver is obviously being exposed to the toxins with each pass. When you are taking Milk Thistle stresses in the liver and semi-interrupts the enterohepatic circuit by interrupting the principal absorption of toxins and by preventing their reabsorption. Cells not yet poisoned are protected from harm from moving toxins and act as stores for the generation of new liver cells. The reason you can recover your liver to new is basically because Milk Thistle also stimulates protein synthesis. Basically, it accelerates the regeneration of damaged liver tissue.

We could go on and on about herbs benefits, providing examples on the way. However, this could be considered a book you are reading and not merely an article. The main stage I need to anxiety about herbs profit is that they are in most cases free to use (just get outside and select them or you can buy them from the store or internet if you do not want to go searching for them), they are cheaper and better than buying manmade drugs, and they've no unwanted effects. Herbs benefits are a thing that we being a society must look much more closely at since rates are merely increasing. This way nobody has to worry about not being able to afford healthcare. Thanks for reading and I hope this has been helpful.

Natural Healing Herbs - The Natural Form of Herb

Vicodin is an analgesic that is quite well known although the world knows it as a painkiller. Allopathic is less prevalent because its remedy involves more time than conventional treatment forms. Now is a big percentage of the world population who would choose natural herbs that heal instead of medicines that heal but have unwanted effects as well. Just about all illnesses may be treated incidentally of herbs. Those activities that are given by nature or all the present herbs allows rewards to individuals with none or less unwanted effects whatsoever.

Devil's claw, is one particular supplement that is renowned in Africa & Europe that has been common for several previous ages and is now finding popularity all across America. This herb has the strength (nothing spiritual whatsoever) where the skeletal system is developed. Studies have reported to it being the same as cortisone. It reduces the brutality of pain in all joints and cells which might be connected to joints.

Pain & insomnia get support via trips. Because it is nutrient rich, the nervous systems receive plenty of the help of trips. The obstructions of spleen & liver are exposed, the blood gets cleaned, from gravel component veins are cleaned, ease the stomach and bursts up urine.

To decrease body nervousness, anxiety and pain hysteria, Passionflower has been demonstrated to be very effective, and that is performed by providing a new lease of life to the nervous system. Through the years Passionflower has been used in both holistic & herbal medications for nervous fatigue, pain, asthma, attention deficit- insomnia & disorder.

Combined and muscle pain comes if you find anxiety and pressure. You can obtain rest from spinal, backache, pain & muscular irritation with quercetin, trace minerals of Coral calcium, sea cucumber extract that guarantees potency and white willow bark.

The brutal consequences of chronic fatigue and the indicators for illustration depression, sore muscles, concentrating troubles, painful joints, anxiety, loss of hunger, frustration, chronic attacks, mood swings, sleep disturbances, muscle soreness, swollen glands, crushing fatigue & memory loss may now he fought with these milk thistle extract, red clover extract, extract of pet's claw, garlic extract, eleuthero extract, ginkgo Biloba extract & gamma-aminobutyric acid (GABA).

Vicodin is recommended in the time of Gout, which can be an unbearable situation. It is a certain arthritis type that occurs due to joints having excessive uric acid.

Vicodin is highly effective for headaches. All of us proceed through a headache all the time, and several of us spend every day experiencing it. In that case, drugs that provide side effects must be stopped. Entirely eliminate them and switch over to herbs which are powerful, they too cure problems and lastly prevent it from arriving again. Herbs assist you in fighting problems via allergies, stress, flow disturbances, sinus infection, environmental toxins, anxiety, temperature, vitamin C, Quercetin, trace minerals having bromelain, coral calcium, cayenne ginkgo Biloba & ninety thousand heat units.

Chapter 3 – Top 7 Tips To Choose Healing Herbs For Your Conditions

Those that use over-the-counter and prescription pharmaceuticals usually know how much medication they are using since FDA regulations require precision. Individuals who use herbs experience more of challenging. However, in controlled amounts, herbs cause fewer side effects than pharmaceuticals. Drugs are highly concentrated, and supplements and capsules have little taste, factors which make it easy to overdose. The active constituents in herbs are usually more distributed, and most style rather sour, which discourages taking too much. When you choose you to wish to use herbs, you are still left with some important issues. Which herbs? And how can you use them? This is a number of popular herbs that are safe and powerful to choose from, along with some information about the circumstances they treat that you can consider.

1. Ephedra

In addition to its decongestant value, Chinese ephedra includes a long history of use in Asia as coffee as a catalyst. New studies have demonstrated that ephedra enhances metabolism - the speed at which calories burn. As a result, it's shown some benefit like a weight-loss support, but just in those who are significantly overweight. Ephedra may also improve heartbeat and blood pressure, so don't utilize it if you have high blood pressure, heart disease, diabetes or glaucoma. If you've thyroid problems, you should not take ephedra. You must discuss it with your doctor if you want to get any product or ephedra containing ephedra.

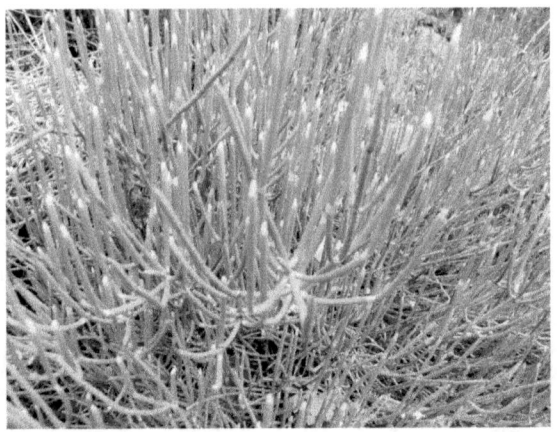

2. Ginseng

Precious above silver for thousands of years, ginseng root continues to be Asia's most revered tonic. It was considered an aphrodisiac that aids longevity enhances health and strengthens the body. Early Jesuit missionaries in Canada created a fortune shipping it to China and found American ginseng in 1704. The supplement was eventually found growing as far south as Georgia, and it quickly became one of the American colonies' most valuable exports, before over collection nearly wiped out it. Today American ginseng is farmed in Wisconsin. Most of the crop is sent to Asia. Data is increasing the herb assists the body resist disease and damage from stress. Studies show that the immune system stimulates, helps lower cholesterol levels, protects the liver from hazardous materials and increases strength and nutrient absorption from the intestines. Asian Olympic athletes go on it regularly to raise their performance.

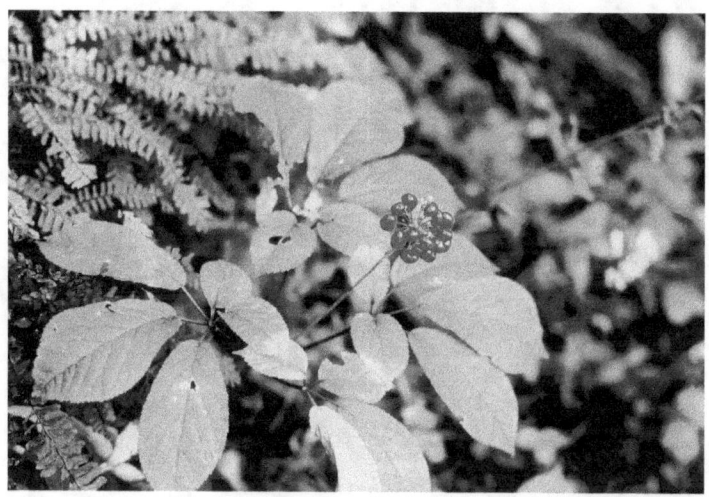

3. Ginger

Scientific research indicates that ginger fights nausea better than anti-nausea drug Dramamine. This root plant does more than simply relieve the stomach. A historical Indian proverb says, "Every good quality is covered in cinnamon." Well, not quite, but studies demonstrate that it also boosts the ability of the immune system to fight infection. And like garlic, it reduces blood pressure and cholesterol and helps prevent the blood clots that trigger a heart attack.

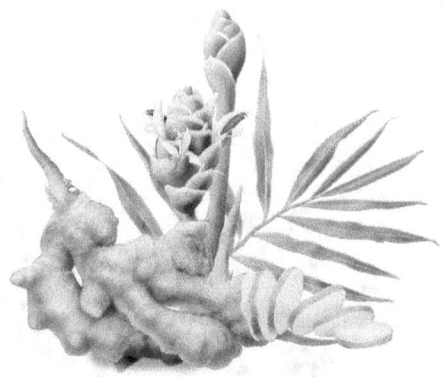

4. Rosemary

A long time before refrigeration was available, the ancients realized that wrap meat in crushed rosemary leaves maintained it and imparted a delicious flavor. Meats ruin in part because oxidation becomes their fats rancid. Rosemary' s chemical action can help prevent food poisoning at your next picnic. Mix the crushed plant into burger meat and tuna, pasta and potato salads. Rosemary also helps relieve the stomach.

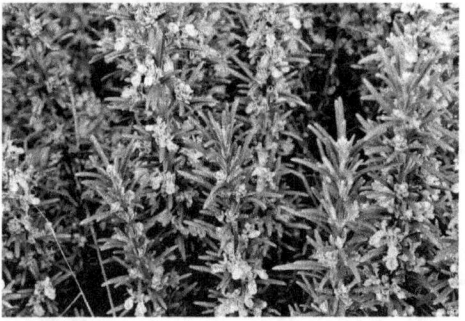

5. Aloe Vera

Throughout the 1930s, the efficiency of aloe Vera was identified by radiologists in treating radiation burns. The latest reports show that the plant has obvious value in treating minor pieces, scrapes, and burns.

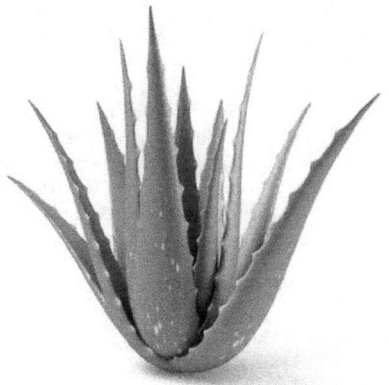

6. Chamomile

When Peter Rabbit got chased out in the wrong end of a hoe and ate himself ill in McGregor's yard, his mom gave him chamomile tea, a traditional therapy for pains, anxiety, and heartburn. Lavender tea is a wonderful home remedy for heartburn, indigestion and infant colic.

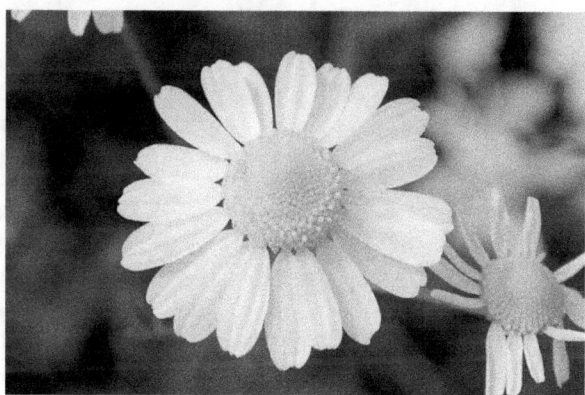

7. Garlic

After ephedra, garlic is considered the world's second oldest medicine. The old world respected garlic as being a virtual panacea, but none liked it as deeply while the Egyptians who consumed so much that the Greek historian Herodotus called them "the stinking ones." Braided garlic flowers put from their doorsteps to keep evil spirits at bay while the centuries passed - a custom echoed today in the garlic braids that adorn many kitchens. During World War I, military doctors employed garlic juice quite effectively to treat wounds and dysentery. Why it worked following the conflict, researchers discovered: When chewed or sliced, garlic is just a powerful natural antibiotic. In fact, five medium cloves pack roughly the exact same antibiotic strike like a common dose of penicillin. Garlic has antiviral properties. Garlic is a good supplement. It will also help lowers and protects against stomach cancer risk of heart disease by reducing cholesterol, lowering blood pressure and decreasing the reality of blood clots that will trigger a heart attack.

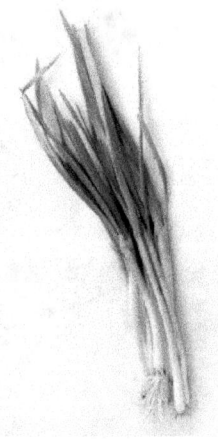

Chapter 5 – The Power of Healing Herbs and Benefits

Modern day women are turning to the healing garden of herbs to treat and prevent issues for example colds, headaches, and allergies, etc. Healing herbs are found right outside your backdoor.

5 Benefits of Healing Herbs:

1. Herbs are a powerful alternative to chemically produced prescriptions or even non-prescription medications. They're able to treat scratches and minor cuts to insomnia and headaches. Herbs provide relief for PMS, indigestion, and even acne. Don't believe of herbs as being a weak substitute to prescriptions as they are powerfully effective.

Instead of applying motion sickness drugs try using Ginger. It is a powerful competitor to perhaps the very best brands sold.

Some studies suggest components from Ginkgo leaves may treat symptoms of Alzheimer's disease.

Of course, it isn't just as replacing conventional medicines with herbal remedies as simple. They ought to work together. Check always with your medical doctor and a seasoned herbalist before mixing herbal treatments with prescription drugs.

2. Making the proper choices and the right dosage will generate fewer negative effects. For your most, part side effects created by herbs are much milder than those produced by drugs. However, you should not take herbal treatments following the need has passed.

For example, if you're going for a prescription for water retention, one complication from your substance will be the destruction of potassium. Around the other hand, the leaves from dandelions not just behave as a diuretic potassium is also supplied by them. Above them, cold remedies may cause drowsiness making it harmful for you to drive or work. Herbs like garlic you can fight off the cold with no drowsy complication.

3. An ounce of elimination is worth a pound of treatment. Reduced immunity pressure, and fatigue weariness all could be decreased with the employment of botanical remedies. Use herbs in cooking and teas for preventive medicine since

some of these might be taken for weeks or weeks without negative effects. This can give minerals and vitamins to your body. Just like any other health plan or diet, you need to incorporate good and exercise eating habits.

4. Herbs are actually suited for the different requirements created by the countless cycles women go through. A female may be supported by herbal remedies through an emotional crisis. Part of the advantages of using herbal remedies will be the simple task of preparing them. Produce beauty products that are beneficial for the body using oils and fragrant herbs. You'll have skincare that'll not reveal you to other ingredients or synthetics.

5. Stop to smell the flowers or the herbs, in this case. The fast pace of life has people operating from one place to another. Small time is left to love the beauty around us. The end of a cup of herbal tea or take an extract of herbs. Enjoying the natural tastes and aromas and reuniting with nature. Start healing yourself emotionally and physically.

Using herbs in even cooking, tinctures, oils and teas is definitely a reward to your health but remember to use organic remedies properly and especially, safely. Generally, herbs are very safe if used in the proper dose. For small medical problems head for the herbs if the situation is more serious go to your physician for a diagnosis. Herbs still could be suitable for treatment or you may combine them under the direction of your doctor with conventional drugs.

Best Healing Herbs for Controlling High Blood Pressure

Having high blood pressure is much like a time bomb. It seldom gives you any symptoms and many people do not even know they've high blood pressure until something happens and they get tested. They wonder how they got high blood pressure. Rest assured; you can use natural herbal remedies to deliver down your blood pressure in a pair of weeks. Keep reading for the record of herbs to use.

Standard blood pressure is approximately 120/80; of course, it depends on each person. Some may have some less count and an increased count. It also depends on age, weight, family history, your lifestyle, and the quantity of stress you've.

Some sign you might have of high blood pressure is nosebleeds, dizzy spells, and headaches. But age is a given, and since most of the people have tension in their lives, you must have your blood pressure tested about once per month to keep tabs on it. Use one of these products in the pharmacy or if the blood bank comes around. Or you can buy a blood pressure system and check it yourself. You can also visit your physician for a blood pressure test. It simply requires a short while, and it could save your life.

To control your high blood pressure with natural healing herbs you need to alter some bad habits. I know, I know, nobody likes changes, but if you wish to stay to a ripe old age, then controlling your blood pressure today may help when you get older.

Below are a few items that need to be taken in moderation.

Find down your weight - the more body you've, the more force there's on your artery walls because more blood is developed to supply oxygen and nutrients to your body. In other words, your weight makes your heart pump harder, and that lifts your blood pressure.

Log off the chair - go for a walk, run in place, chase your family members around the house, walk or run upstairs, jog out to the address, do some jumping jacks, jump up and down, do something, anything to get more action. Lack of physical activity improves the causes and your heart rate your heart to pump harder, again raising your blood pressure.

Cut the salt - excessive salt in water retention and high blood pressure in your diet effects. They put or sodium in our food supply as a chemical; you do not really need any more. Or better yet, stop eat prepared meals - eat fresh ingredients like vegetables, fruits, and nuts.

Find your potassium - low potassium results in increased sodium (salt) in cells. You need potassium to balance the sodium in your body. Eat a banana a day; try eating avocados a few times weekly; fresh apricots, cantaloupe, honeydew, kiwi, lima beans (yuk!) but good for you and dairy, prunes, spinach, apples, oranges, tomatoes and winter squashes all contain potassium in amounts you need daily. Cannot handle some of them? Then create a smoothie and drink it on the run, but make use of the whole fruit or plant, not merely the juice. Also, do not forget to eat your beef, poultry, and fish.

Things to keep to a minimum - alcohol, cigarette, and stress. Over time, high blood pressure will be caused by all these products, so try to maintain their use to a minimum. Excessive consumption of these products -- the higher your blood pressure will get. The keyword is Excessive. Maintain the utilization of these to a minimum. And try not to pressure over every little thing. Choose your stress properly.

Age - little you may do about this until you have a stasis chamber to use every night. Be gentle on your body and it'll last a lifetime.

Water - the pillar of the body. The more water you consume the faster, it reduces the unwelcome out of your body. Yes, eight glasses of water each day could make you pee a lot, but this is the point. It wipes out the terrible from your body. Try drinking eight glasses of water for monthly and see if you do not feel better. You'll be amazed at the difference.

Today for the natural herbal remedies for high blood pressure:

1. Garlic – Garlic is something which comes in mind 1st while thinking of the body feel better. Garlic not just lowers high blood pressure. However, it also increases low blood pressure. It is similar to a blood pressure regulator. It's up to you, but

using fresh garlic is a lot better for you than using garlic supplements. Garlic products are inferior and completely useless.

Use 3 to 5 cloves a day for maximum benefit. Make some garlic butter and wear your toast in the day, combine it with mayonnaise for salad, set it in sauces and sauté it with any beef or place it in with a vegetable or fruit smoothie.

2. Flax seed. Many people don't know the uses of flaxseed, but it contains omega 3, which really is a fatty acid (one the body needs), the same form that's in fish and the same type that will lower your blood pressure. I am not really a big fan of products, so I use flaxseed whole and make what I need. It's such a wide range of uses, and one is to reduce your blood pressure.

Use one teaspoon per cup of water. Hard boil for 3 minutes, appreciate your flax seed tea, stress the vegetables and cool slightly. It gets a little solid when it cools, so it's best to drink it hot. Have 1 to 3 cup per day for fourteen days and you will see your blood pressure drop. You and more than three cups I'll be managing to the bathroom far more. It might, with respect to the person, behave as a laxative if too much is taken. So beware!

3. Cayenne is employed for circulation. Yes, they are hot, but this is the place. It helps sweat out the toxins in your body and forces the body to move the blood. The source of the warmth is capsaicin, the hot resin located in hottest peppers. Capsaicin causes nerve endings to produce a substance called substance P. Substance P sends pain signals from your body back to the brain.

It's also good for the entire digestive system. It operates as a driver and increases the success of other herbs. It's a very high source of Vitamins A and D, has the complete b-complexes, and is extremely rich in organic calcium and potassium; that is one of the reasons why it is great for your heart.

Utilize a couple of fresh cayenne or any hot peppers every day to get the total benefits of the amazing little herbs. They taste good with eggs in the morning. If you don't preserve, then a couple of capsules a day will get you the same benefits.

4. - Hawthorn must true be number 2 before I use hawthorn but I like flaxseed. Hawthorn is employed to protect against initial phases of high blood pressure and heart disease. Using the flowers, leaves, and fruits all help to start the arteries and improving blood flow, softening deposits (material in your arteries), and makes a superb remedy for angina. It decides heart irregularities and will calm an over-rapid heart rate.

Reducer of High Blood Pressure Tea

1-quart boiling water

1 teaspoon each hawthorn fruits and plants, ginger rhizome, valerian root and motherwort leaves

Pour over extreme and the herbs for 20 minutes. Strain herbs. Drink at least 2 cups each day. Utilizing the same proportions, you may also make these herbs into a tincture, or you can get a commercial tincture only at the herb shop. Furthermore, you can also use supplements and pills.

As with all assistance, check with your physician before mixing and related herbs with treatment. To see why your blood pressure is so high. Using healing herbs won't support if you keep doing what creating your high blood pressure. Learn why then use these herbal remedies to bring it under control.

In our nights there are less and fewer individuals who believe in their capabilities, although some of the countries have been using healing herbs for thousands of years. Though you mightn't think of them, you may still see the consequences that they have.

Garlic

That is one of the healing herbs and spices that is typically used for seasoning. Nonetheless, it may also be used for reducing the cholesterol levels, it may not combat hot, and it reduces high blood pressure.

Ginger

Specific herbs and herbs possess a more exotic style, and ginger is one of them. Even so, some people use it to treat nausea and an upset stomach. The other properties of ginger include antibacterial, anti- inflammatory and antiviral properties.

Sage

Sage also belongs to the herbs and spices that are utilized for filling and seasoning, but it can perform more than that. It generally induces a feeling of a clear head, fulfillment and it can also be utilized to prevent memory loss that comes with age.

Turmeric

From India, a whole lot of spices and herbs have been added in the past, and this can be one of them. It's helpful for the liver, and it creates fat burn faster, promoting weight loss. In the case of gallbladder and eye diseases, it can benefit besides all of this.

Cinnamon

Cinnamon is usually used in case of coffee, teas, French toast and even pastries. Besides this, just like a number of other herbs and spices it can benefit diabetics remove spikes in the blood sugar after eating.

Aloe

That is one of the most well-known healing herbs. Generally, it's used for treating sunburn, scratches, scalds, and burns and it is recognized for being an infection fighter. Also, manufacturers use it in cosmetics to make the skin prettier.

Basil

A whole lot of healing herbs have already been used as seasoning also, and only some people know that basil can be used to treat organisms, acne and also for stimulating the immune system.

Chamomile

Some of the healing herbs can be used for nearly every problem, and lavender is one of them. It can treat ulcers and injuries and also inflammations and indigestions. Menstrual cramps can be treated with it and well as arthritis, and it's a sedative effect.

Eucalyptus

That is one of the healing herbs which were used in candy for loosening phlegm, and it also kills flu.

Conclusion

Effective healing herbs do exist alternatively; you only need to know how to use them and where to get the right herbs.

How to Find Herbs

You can grow many of them yourself, or you can select up them even or at local herbal health food stores on the Internet. You'll find them available in several common types if you're buying them. These include floor powder to make tinctures, tea, or oil components or tablets. It is often important to examine the strength of healing herbs before you buy them, to ensure performance and safety. You should always be certain that the herbal health food store you are buying from can be a respectable source that could grow and process its herbs correctly before selling to the buyer. If you are an initial time buyer, contact the store, and ask for their information about how they handle their herbs, etc. Stores that will not disclose this kind of information should be avoided.

What to Do with Herbs

Many therapeutic herbs already exist in industry today, often incorporated into other products. Firms have realized the fact that healing herbs have become popular, so for example, herbs like aloe Vera are often being added to face products and even suntan lotions.